Plant-Based Salads for Women Over 60

Complete Vegetarian Meals to Power Your Day

By Rollo McCain

Sommario

INTRODUCTION

Many people consider vegetarianism as a lifestyle that in addition to respecting animals also has other important advantages such as a great reduction in the risk of chronic diseases and diabetes. mainly they are divided into two strands, in fact there are some of them who prefer to consume at least products of animal origin and others who, instead, taking their beliefs to the extreme, prefer to eliminate even those and are called vegans. in both cases the choice is made to abolish all forms of meat including chicken, beef, game and fish. At this point I recommend that you go in search of your favorite dish in our fantastic book, Bon Appetite.

SALADS

Butter Lettuce Onion and Tarragon Salad

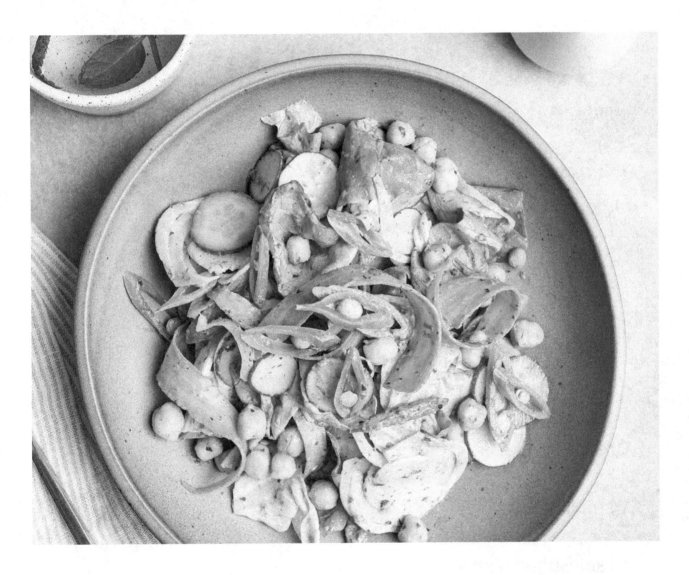

Ingredients:

3 ounces cream cheese, crumbled

3 ounces mozarella cheese,
shredded 3 ounces parmesan

cheese, shredded

6 to 7 cups Butter lettuce, 3 bundles, trimmed

1/4 European or seedless cucumber, halved lengthwise, then thinlysliced

3 tablespoons chopped or snipped chives16 cherry tomatoes

1/2 cup sliced almonds1/4 white onion, sliced

2 to 3 tablespoons chopped tarragon leavesSalt and pepper, to taste

Dressing

1 small shallot, minced

1 tablespoon distilled white vinegar 1/4 lemon, juiced, about 2 teaspoons1/4 cup extra-virgin olive oil

Prep

Combine all of the dressing ingredients in a food processor. Toss with the rest of the ingredients and combine well.

Romaine Lettuce Tomatoes Almond and Tarragon Salad

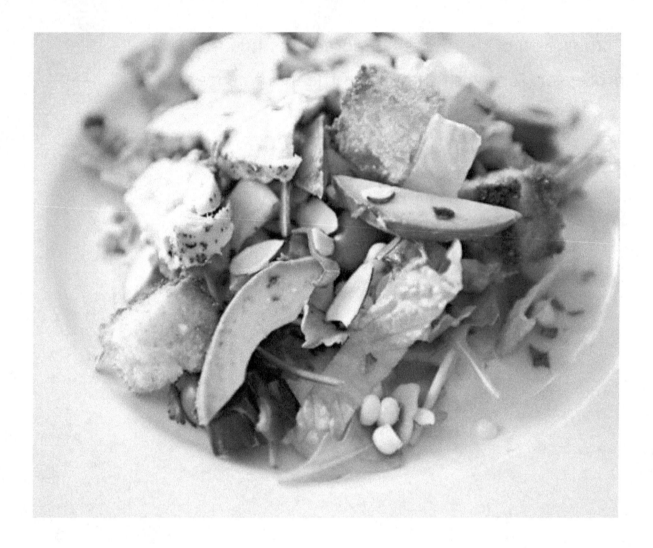

Ingredients:

3 ounces pecorino romano cheese,
shredded3 ounces cream cheese,
crumbled

3 ounces mozarella cheese, shredded

6 to 7 cups Romaine lettuce, 3 bundles, trimmed

1/4 European or seedless cucumber, halved lengthwise, then thinly sliced

3 tablespoons chopped or snipped chives 16 cherry tomatoes

1/2 cup sliced almonds 1/4 white onion, sliced

2 to 3 tablespoons chopped tarragon leaves Salt and pepper, to taste

Dressing

1 small shallot, minced

1 tablespoon distilled white vinegar 1/4 lemon, juiced, about 2 teaspoons 1/4 cup extra-virgin olive oil

Prep

Combine all of the dressing ingredients in a food

processor. Toss with the rest of the ingredients and combine well.

Romaine Tomatoes with Cream Cheese and Hazelnut Salad

Ingredients:

3 ounces monterey jack cheese, shredded 3 ounces ricotta cheese

3 ounces cheddar cheese , shredded

6 to 7 cups Romaine lettuce, 3 bundles, trimmed

1/4 European or seedless cucumber, halved lengthwise, then thinly sliced

3 tablespoons chopped or snipped chives 16 cherry tomatoes

1/2 cup sliced hazelnuts 1/4 white onion, sliced

2 to 3 tablespoons chopped tarragon leaves Salt and pepper, to taste

Dressing

1 small shallot, minced

1 tablespoon distilled white
vinegar 1/4 lemon, juiced, about 2
teaspoons 1/4 cup extra-virgin
olive oil

Prep

Combine all of the dressing ingredients in a food
processor. Toss with the rest of the ingredients and
combine well.

Butter Lettuce and Zucchini with Parmesan Salad

Ingredients:

5 ounces cream cheese, crumbled

3 ounces mozarella cheese,
shredded1 ounces parmesan
cheese, shredded

6 to 7 cups Butter lettuce, 3 bundles, trimmed

1/4 Zucchini, halved lengthwise, then thinly
sliced16 cherry tomatoes

1/2 cup sliced
almonds1/4 white
onion, sliced

2 to 3 tablespoons chopped tarragon
leavesSalt and pepper, to taste

Dressing

1 small shallot, minced

1 tablespoon distilled white
vinegar 1/4 lemon, juiced, about 2
teaspoons 1/4 cup extra-virgin
olive oil

Prep

Combine all of the dressing ingredients in a food
processor. Toss with the rest of the ingredients and
combine well.

Romaine Lettuce with Mozarella and Hazelnut Salad

Ingredients:

6 ounces mozarella cheese,
shredded3 ounces parmesan
cheese, shredded

6 to 7 cups Romaine lettuce, 3 bundles, trimmed

1/4 European or seedless cucumber, halved lengthwise, then
thinlysliced

3 tablespoons chopped or snipped
chives16 cherry tomatoes

1/2 cup sliced
hazelnuts1/4 white
onion, sliced

2 to 3 tablespoons chopped tarragon
leavesSalt and pepper, to taste

Dressing

1 small shallot, minced

1 tablespoon distilled white
vinegar 1/4 lemon, juiced, about 2
teaspoons 1/4 cup extra-virgin
olive oil

Prep

Combine all of the dressing ingredients in a food
processor. Toss with the rest of the ingredients and
combine well.

Iceberg Lettuce Tomatoes Mozarella and Almond Salad

Ingredients:

3 ounces cream cheese, crumbled

5 ounces mozarella cheese, shredded

6 to 7 cups Iceberg lettuce, 3 bundles, trimmed

1/4 European or seedless cucumber, halved lengthwise, then thinlysliced

3 tablespoons chopped or snipped
chives16 cherry tomatoes

1/2 cup sliced
almonds1/4 white
onion, sliced

2 to 3 tablespoons chopped tarragon
leavesSalt and pepper, to taste

Dressing

1 small shallot, minced

1 tablespoon distilled white
vinegar 1/4 lemon, juiced, about 2
teaspoons 1/4 cup extra-virgin
olive oil

Prep

Combine all of the dressing ingredients in a food
processor. Toss with the rest of the ingredients and
combine well.

Romaine Lettuce Cream Cheese and Pistachio Salad

Ingredients:

5 ounces cream cheese, crumbled

3 ounces mozarella cheese, shredded

6 to 7 cups Romaine lettuce, 3 bundles, trimmed

1/4 European or seedless cucumber, halved lengthwise, then thinlysliced

3 tablespoons chopped or snipped
chives16 cherry tomatoes

1/2 cup sliced
pistachios1/4 Vidalla
onion, sliced

2 to 3 tablespoons chopped tarragon
leavesSalt and pepper, to taste

Dressing

1 small shallot, minced

1 tablespoon distilled white
vinegar 1/4 lemon, juiced, about 2
teaspoons 1/4 cup extra-virgin
olive oil

Prep

Combine all of the dressing ingredients in a food
processor. Toss with the rest of the ingredients and
combine well.

Frisee Mozarella and Feta Salad

Ingredients:

6 to 7 cups butter head lettuce, 3 bundles, trimmed

1/4 seedless cucumber, halved lengthwise, then thinly sliced3 tablespoons chopped or snipped chives

16 cherry tomatoes1/2 cup pistachios

1/4 white onion, sliced

2 to 3 tablespoons chopped tarragon leavesSalt and pepper, to taste

3 ounces mozarella cheese, shredded6 ounces parmesan cheese, shredded

Dressing

1 small shallot, minced

1 tablespoon distilled white
vinegar 1/4 lemon, juiced, about 2
teaspoons1/4 cup extra-virgin
olive oil

1 tbsp. pesto sauce

Prep

Combine all of the dressing ingredients in a food
processor. Toss with the rest of the ingredients and
combine well.

Romaine Lettuce with Pepperjack and Feta Salad

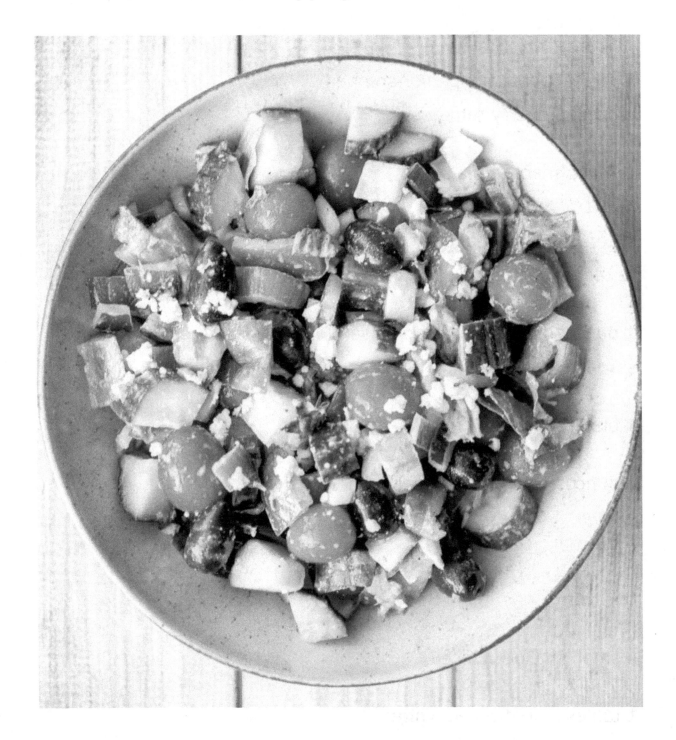

Ingredients:

6 to 7 cups romaine lettuce, 3 bundles, trimmed

1/4 European or seedless cucumber, halved lengthwise, then thinlysliced

3 tablespoons chopped or snipped chives16 cherry tomatoes

1/2 cup macadamia nuts1/4 red onion, sliced Salt and pepper, to taste

1 ounces monterey jack cheese, shredded3 ounces ricotta cheese

1 ounces cheddar cheese , shredded

1 ounces pepperjack cheese, shredded

Dressing

1 small shallot, minced

1 tablespoon distilled white vinegar 1/4 lemon, juiced, about 2 teaspoons1/4 cup extra-virgin olive oil

1 tbsp. pesto sauce

Prep

Combine all of the dressing ingredients in a food processor. Toss with the rest of the ingredients and combine well.

Loose-leaf Lettuce Tomato and 4 Cheese Salad

Ingredients:

6 to 7 cups loose leaf lettuce, 3 bundles, trimmed 1/4 cucumber, halved lengthwise, then thinly sliced16 cherry tomatoes

1/4 red onion, sliced

2 to 3 tablespoons chopped fresh basilSalt and pepper, to taste

2 ounces cheddar cheese , shredded

2 ounces pepperjack cheese, shredded

3 ounces pecorino romano cheese, shredded2 ounces cream cheese, crumbled

Dressing

1 small shallot, minced

1 tablespoon distilled white

vinegar 1/4 lemon, juiced, about 2
teaspoons 1/4 cup extra-virgin
olive oil

Prep

Combine all of the dressing ingredients in a food
processor. Toss with the rest of the ingredients and
combine well.

Frisee Lettuce Tomatoes and Pecorino Romano

Ingredients:

6 to 7 cups frisee lettuce, 3 bundles, trimmed

1/4 cucumber, halved lengthwise, then thinly
sliced 3 tablespoons chopped or snipped chives

16 cherry tomatoes
1/2 cup sliced
almonds 1/4 red
onion, sliced

2 to 3 tablespoons chopped
parsley Salt and pepper, to taste

3 ounces ricotta cheese

2 ounces cheddar cheese , shredded

1 ounces pepperjack cheese, shredded

1 ounces pecorino romano cheese, shredded

Dressing

1 small scallions, minced

1 tablespoon distilled white
vinegar 1/4 lemon, juiced, about
2 teaspoons 1/4 cup macadamia
nut oil

Prep

Combine all of the dressing ingredients in a food
processor. Toss with the rest of the ingredients and
combine well.

Romaine Lettuce Tomatoes and Ricotta

Ingredients:

2 ounces monterey jack cheese,
shredded2 ounces ricotta cheese

2 ounces cheddar cheese , shredded

2 ounces pepperjack cheese, shredded

6 to 7 cups romaine lettuce, 3 bundles, trimmed

1/4 European or seedless cucumber, halved lengthwise, then thinlysliced

3 tablespoons chopped or snipped
chives16 cherry tomatoes

1/2 cup pistachios
1/4 red onion,
sliced

Salt and pepper, to taste

Dressing

1 small shallot, minced

1 tablespoon distilled white
vinegar 1/4 lemon, juiced, about 2
teaspoons1/4 cup extra-virgin
olive oil

Prep

Combine all of the dressing ingredients in a food
processor.Toss with the rest of the ingredients and
combine well.

Loose-leaf Lettuce and Pecorino Romano Salad

Ingredients:

3 ounces pepperjack cheese, shredded

3 ounces pecorino romano cheese,
shredded 3 ounces cream cheese,
crumbled

3 ounces mozarella cheese, shredded

6 to 7 cups loose leaf head lettuce, 3 bundles,
trimmed 1/4 cucumber, halved lengthwise, then
thinly sliced

3 tablespoons snipped
chives 16 cherry tomatoes

1/2 cup peanuts

1/4 white onion, sliced
Salt and pepper, to
taste

Dressing

1 small shallot, minced

2 tablespoon distilled white vinegar1/4 cup sesame seed oil

1 tbsp. Thai chili garlic sauce

Prep

Combine all of the dressing ingredients in a food processor. Toss with the rest of the ingredients and combine well.

Butterhead Chives and Pistachio Salad

Ingredients:

7 cups loose butterhead lettuce, 3 bundles, trimmed

1/4 European or seedless cucumber, halved lengthwise, then thinlysliced

3 tablespoons chopped or snipped chives16 grapes

1/2 cup
pistachios1/4
onion, sliced

Salt and pepper, to
taste6 ounces vegan
cheese

Dressing

1 sprig parsley, chopped

1 tablespoon distilled white

vinegar 1/4 lemon, juiced, about 2
teaspoons 1/4 cup extra-virgin
olive oil

Prep

Combine all of the dressing ingredients in a food
processor. Toss with the rest of the ingredients and
combine well.

Boston Lettuce Almond and Vegan Cream Cheese Salad

Ingredients:

7 cups Boston lettuce, 3 bundles, trimmed

½ cucumber, halved lengthwise, then thinly
sliced 3 tablespoons chopped or snipped
chives

16 cherry tomatoes
1/2 cup sliced
almonds 1/4 red
onion, sliced

Salt and pepper, to taste

7 ounces vegan cream cheese

Dressing

1 small shallot, minced

1 tablespoon distilled white
vinegar 1/4 lemon, juiced, about 2

teaspoons1/4 cup extra-virgin olive oil

1 tbsp. chimichurri sauce

Prep

Combine all of the dressing ingredients in a food processor. Toss with the rest of the ingredients and combine well.

Frisee Lettuce and Tomato Salad d

Ingredients:

6 to 7 cups Frisee lettuce, 3 bundles, trimmed

1/4 cucumber, halved lengthwise, then thinly
sliced3 tablespoons chopped or snipped chives

16 cherry tomatoes

1/2 cup sliced

almonds1/4 red

onion, sliced

Salt and pepper, to taste

3 ounces pepperjack cheese, shredded

3 ounces pecorino romano cheese,

shredded3 ounces cream cheese,

crumbled

3 ounces mozarella cheese, shredded

Dressing

1 sprig parsley, minced

1 tablespoon distilled white
vinegar 1/4 lemon, juiced, about 2
teaspoons 1/4 cup extra-virgin
olive oil

Prep

Combine all of the dressing ingredients in a food
processor. Toss with the rest of the ingredients and
combine well.

Mesclun and Tomato with Cilantro Vinaigrette

Ingredients:

6 to 7 cups mesclun, 3 bundles, trimmed

1/4 cucumber, halved lengthwise, then thinly
sliced 3 tablespoons chopped or snipped chives

16 cherry tomatoes

1/2 cup sliced

almonds 1/4 white

onion, sliced

Salt and pepper, to taste

1 ounce blue cheese, crumbled

3 ounces gouda cheese,

shredded 3 ounces brie cheese,

crumbled

Dressing

1 sprig cilantro, minced

1 tablespoon distilled white
vinegar 1/4 lemon, juiced, about 2
teaspoons1/4 cup extra-virgin
olive oil

Prep

Combine all of the dressing ingredients in a food
processor. Toss with the rest of the ingredients and
combine well.

Chervil and Almond Salad

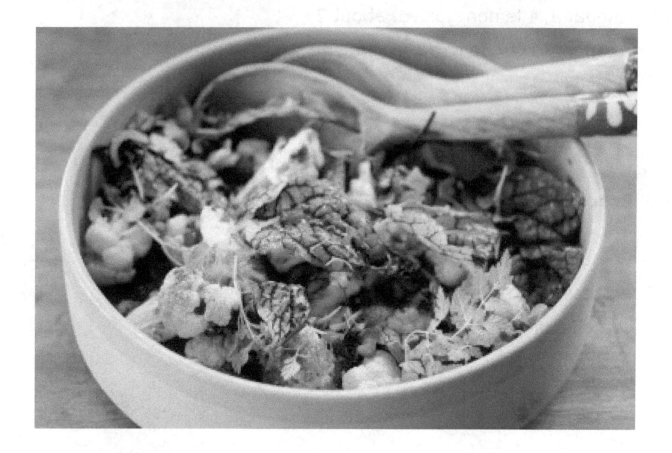

Ingredients:

7 cups chervil, 3 bundles, trimmed

1/4 cucumber, halved lengthwise, then thinly
sliced 3 tablespoons chopped or snipped chives

16 cherry tomatoes
1/2 cup sliced
almonds 1/4 white
onion, sliced

Salt and pepper, to taste

3 ounces parmesan cheese,
shredded1 ounce blue cheese,
crumbled

3 ounces gouda cheese, shredded

Dressing

1 tablespoon distilled white
vinegar 1/4 lemon, juiced, about 2
teaspoons1/4 cup extra-virgin
olive oil

1 tsp. English mustard

Prep

Combine all of the dressing ingredients in a food
processor.Toss with the rest of the ingredients and
combine well.

Bib Lettuce and Vegan Ricotta Salad

Ingredients:

6 to 7 cups bib lettuce, 3 bundles, trimmed

1/4 cucumber, halved lengthwise, then thinly sliced 16 grapes

1/2 cup sliced almonds
1/4 white onion, sliced
Salt and pepper, to
taste

3 ounces mozarella cheese, shredded 3 ounces parmesan cheese, shredded 1 ounce blue cheese, crumbled

Dressing

1 tablespoon distilled white vinegar 1/4 lemon, juiced, about 2 teaspoons 1/4 cup extra-virgin olive oil

1 tbsp. Chimichurri sauce

Prep

Combine all of the dressing ingredients in a food processor. Toss with the rest of the ingredients and combine well.

Boston Lettuce Walnut and Vegan Parmesan Salad

Ingredients:

6 to 7 cups boston lettuce, 3 bundles, trimmed

1/4 cucumber, halved lengthwise, then thinly
sliced 3 tablespoons chopped or snipped chives

16 tomatillos, sliced in
half 1/2 cup walnuts

1/4 red onion, sliced
Salt and pepper, to
taste

3 ounces camembert cheese,
crumbled 3 ounces mozarella cheese,
shredded 3 ounces parmesan
cheese, shredded

Dressing

1 tablespoon distilled white
vinegar 1/4 lemon, juiced, about 2

teaspoons 1/4 cup extra-virgin olive oil

1 tsp. egg free mayonnaise

Prep

Combine all of the dressing ingredients in a food processor. Toss with the rest of the ingredients and combine well.

Endive Lettuce Tomatillo and Vegan Ricotta Salad

Ingredients:

6 to 7 cups endive, 3 bundles, trimmed

1/4 cucumber, halved lengthwise, then thinly
sliced3 tablespoons chopped or snipped chives

16 green tomatillos, sliced in
half1/2 cup sliced almonds

1/4 white onion, sliced
Salt and pepper, to
taste

3 ounces pecorino romano cheese,
shredded3 ounces cream cheese,
crumbled

3 ounces camembert cheese, crumbled

Dressing

1 tablespoon distilled white

vinegar 1/4 lemon, juiced, about 2
teaspoons 1/4 cup extra-virgin
olive oil

1 tsp. Dijon mustard

Prep

Combine all of the dressing ingredients in a food
processor. Toss with the rest of the ingredients and
combine well.

Kale Tomato and Vegan Parmesan Salad

Ingredients:

6 to 7 cups kale, 3 bundles, trimmed

1/4 cucumber, halved lengthwise, then thinly
sliced 3 tablespoons chopped or snipped chives

16 cherry tomatoes

1/2 cup sliced

almonds 1/4 white

onion, sliced

Salt and pepper, to taste

3 ounces pepperjack cheese, shredded

3 ounces pecorino romano cheese,
shredded 3 ounces cream cheese,
crumbled

Dressing

1 sprig cilantro, minced

1 tablespoon distilled white
vinegar 1/4 lemon, juiced, about 2
teaspoons 1/4 cup extra-virgin
olive oil

1 tsp. egg free mayonnaise

Prep

Combine all of the dressing ingredients in a food
processor. Toss with the rest of the ingredients and
combine well.

Lettuce Tomatillos and Almond Salad

Ingredients:

6 to 7 cups lettuce, 3 bundles, trimmed

1/4 cucumber, halved lengthwise, then thinly
sliced3 tablespoons chopped or snipped chives

16 tomatillos, sliced in
half1/2 cup sliced
almonds 1/4 white
onion, sliced Salt and
pepper, to taste

3 ounces cream cheese, crumbled

3 ounces camembert cheese,
crumbled3 ounces mozarella cheese,
shredded

Dressing

1 sprig cilantro, minced

1 tablespoon distilled white
vinegar 1/4 lemon, juiced, about 2
teaspoons 1/4 cup extra-virgin
olive oil

1 tsp. English mustard

Prep

Combine all of the dressing ingredients in a food
processor. Toss with the rest of the ingredients and
combine well.

Kale Tomato and Almond Salad

Ingredients:

6 to 7 cups kale, 3 bundles, trimmed

1/4 cucumber, halved lengthwise, then thinly
sliced 3 tablespoons chopped or snipped chives

16 cherry tomatoes
1/2 cup sliced
almonds 1/4 white
onion, sliced

Salt and pepper, to taste

3 ounces camembert cheese,
crumbled 3 ounces mozarella cheese,
shredded 3 ounces parmesan
cheese, shredded

Dressing

1 sprig cilantro, minced

1 tablespoon distilled white
vinegar 1/4 lemon, juiced, about 2
teaspoons 1/4 cup extra-virgin
olive oil

1 tsp. English mustard

Prep

Combine all of the dressing ingredients in a food
processor. Toss with the rest of the ingredients and
combine well.

Kale Almond and Vegan Ricotta Salad

Ingredients:

6 to 7 cups kale, 3 bundles, trimmed

1/4 cucumber, halved lengthwise, then thinly
sliced3 tablespoons chopped or snipped chives

16 green tomatillos, sliced in
half1/2 cup sliced almonds

1/4 white onion, sliced
Salt and pepper, to
taste

3 ounces cottage cheese, crumbled

3 ounces pepperjack cheese, shredded

3 ounces pecorino romano cheese, shredded

Dressing

1 tablespoon distilled white
vinegar 1/4 lemon, juiced, about 2

teaspoons1/4 cup extra-virgin
olive oil

1 tsp. Dijon mustard

Prep

Combine all of the dressing ingredients in a food
processor. Toss with the rest of the ingredients and
combine well.

Escarole Tomato and Almond Salad

Ingredients:

6 to 7 cups escarole, 3 bundles, trimmed

1/4 cucumber, halved lengthwise, then thinly
sliced3 tablespoons chopped or snipped chives

16 cherry tomatoes
1/2 cup sliced
almonds1/4 white
onion, sliced

Salt and pepper, to
taste3 ounces ricotta
cheese

3 ounces cheddar cheese ,
shredded3 ounces cottage cheese,
crumbled

Dressing

1 sprig cilantro, minced

1 tablespoon distilled white
vinegar 1/4 lemon, juiced, about 2
teaspoons 1/4 cup extra-virgin
olive oil

1 tsp. English mustard

Prep

Combine all of the dressing ingredients in a food
processor. Toss with the rest of the ingredients and
combine well.

Mesclun Tomatillo and Almond Salad

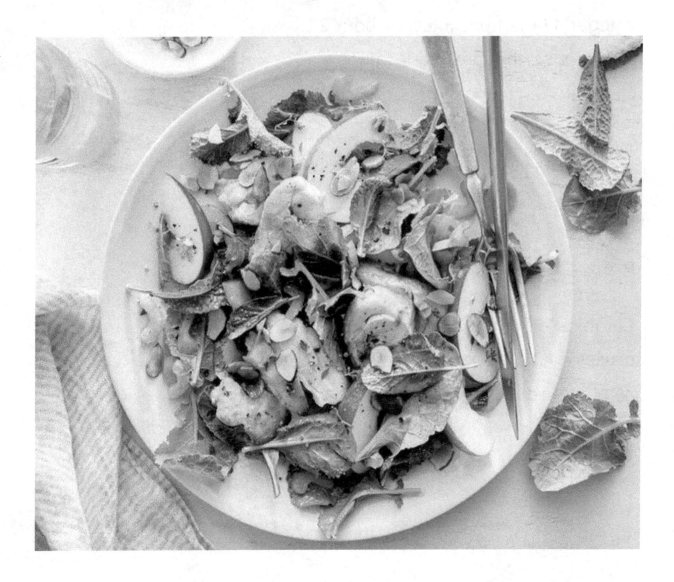

Ingredients:

6 to 7 cups mesclun, 3 bundles, trimmed

1/4 cucumber, halved lengthwise, then thinly
sliced 3 tablespoons chopped or snipped chives

16 tomatillos, sliced in
half 1/2 cup sliced

almonds 1/4 white
onion, sliced Salt and
pepper, to taste

3 ounces feta cheese,
crumbled 3 ounces ricotta
cheese

3 ounces cheddar cheese , shredded

Dressing

1 tablespoon distilled white
vinegar 1/4 lemon, juiced, about 2
teaspoons 1/4 cup extra-virgin
olive oil

1 tsp. egg-free mayonnaise

Prep

Combine all of the dressing ingredients in a food
processor. Toss with the rest of the ingredients and
combine well.

Endive Almond and Tomato Salad

Ingredients:

6 to 7 cups endive, 3 bundles, trimmed

1/4 cucumber, halved lengthwise, then thinly
sliced 3 tablespoons chopped or snipped chives

16 cherry tomatoes
1/2 cup sliced
almonds 1/4 white
onion, sliced

Salt and pepper, to taste

3 ounces cheddar cheese ,
shredded 3 ounces cottage cheese,
crumbled

3 ounces pepperjack cheese, shredded

Dressing

1 sprig cilantro, minced

1 tablespoon distilled white
vinegar 1/4 lemon, juiced, about 2
teaspoons1/4 cup extra-virgin
olive oil

1 tsp. English mustard

Prep

Combine all of the dressing ingredients in a food
processor. Toss with the rest of the ingredients and
combine well.

Bib Lettuce Tomatillo and Almond Salad

Ingredients:

6 to 7 cups bib lettuce, 3 bundles, trimmed

1/4 cucumber, halved lengthwise, then thinly sliced3 tablespoons chopped or snipped chives

16 tomatillos, sliced in half1/2 cup sliced almonds 1/4 white onion, sliced Salt and pepper, to taste

3 ounces monterey jack cheese, shredded3 ounces feta cheese, crumbled

3 ounces ricotta cheese**Dressing**

1 tablespoon distilled white vinegar 1/4 lemon, juiced, about 2 teaspoons1/4 cup extra-virgin olive oil

1 tsp. Dijon mustard

Prep

Combine all of the dressing ingredients in a food processor. Toss with the rest of the ingredients and combine well.

Endives Almond and Cherry Tomato Salad

Ingredients:

6 to 7 cups endives, 3 bundles, trimmed

1/4 cucumber, halved lengthwise, then thinly sliced3 tablespoons chopped or snipped chives

16 cherry tomatoes

1/2 cup sliced

almonds1/4 white

onion, sliced

Salt and pepper, to taste

3 ounces feta cheese,

crumbled3 ounces ricotta

cheese

Dressing

1 sprig cilantro, minced

1 tablespoon distilled white

vinegar 1/4 lemon, juiced, about 2
teaspoons 1/4 cup extra-virgin
olive oil

1 tsp. English mustard

Prep

Combine all of the dressing ingredients in a food
processor. Toss with the rest of the ingredients and
combine well.

Butter Lettuce and Feta Cheese Salad

Ingredients:

6 to 7 cups butter lettuce, 3 bundles, trimmed

1/4 cucumber, halved lengthwise, then thinly
sliced 3 tablespoons chopped or snipped chives

16 tomatillos, sliced in
half 1/2 cup sliced
almonds 1/4 white
onion, sliced Salt and
pepper, to taste

6 ounces monterey jack cheese,
shredded 3 ounces feta cheese,
crumbled

Dressing

1 sprig cilantro, minced

1 tablespoon distilled white
vinegar 1/4 lemon, juiced, about 2

teaspoons 1/4 cup extra-virgin olive oil

1 tsp. egg free mayonnaise

Prep

Combine all of the dressing ingredients in a food processor. Toss with the rest of the ingredients and combine well.

Kale Tomato and Ricotta Cheese Salad

Ingredients:

6 to 7 cups kale lettuce, 3 bundles, trimmed

1/4 cucumber, halved lengthwise, then thinly
sliced 3 tablespoons chopped or snipped chives

16 cherry tomatoes
1/2 cup sliced
almonds 1/4 white
onion, sliced

Salt and pepper, to taste

3 ounces feta cheese,
crumbled 5 ounces ricotta
cheese

Dressing

1 sprig cilantro, minced

1 tablespoon distilled white

vinegar 1/4 lemon, juiced, about 2
teaspoons 1/4 cup extra-virgin
olive oil

1 tsp. English mustard

Prep

Combine all of the dressing ingredients in a food
processor. Toss with the rest of the ingredients and
combine well.

Mesclun Tomatillo and Cottage Cheese Salad

Ingredients:

6 to 7 cups mesclun, 3 bundles, trimmed

1/4 cucumber, halved lengthwise, then thinly
sliced 3 tablespoons chopped or snipped chives

16 green tomatillos, sliced in
half 1/2 cup sliced almonds

1/4 white onion, sliced
Salt and pepper, to
taste

5 ounces cottage cheese, crumbled

3 ounces pepperjack cheese, shredded

Dressing

1 sprig cilantro, minced

1 tablespoon distilled white
vinegar 1/4 lemon, juiced, about 2

teaspoons 1/4 cup extra-virgin
olive oil

Prep

Combine all of the dressing ingredients in a food
processor. Toss with the rest of the ingredients and
combine well.

Escarole Almond and Vegan Ricotta Cheese Salad

Ingredients:

6 to 7 cups escarole, 3 bundles, trimmed

1/4 cucumber, halved lengthwise, then thinly
sliced3 tablespoons chopped or snipped chives

16 tomatillos, sliced in
half1/2 cup sliced
almonds 1/4 white
onion, sliced Salt and
pepper, to taste

3 ounces cheddar cheese ,
shredded3 ounces cottage cheese,
crumbled

Dressing

1 tablespoon distilled white
vinegar 1/4 lemon, juiced, about 2
teaspoons1/4 cup extra-virgin
olive oil

1 tsp. Dijon mustard

Prep

Combine all of the dressing ingredients in a food processor. Toss with the rest of the ingredients and combine well.

Endive Tomato and Ricotta Cheese Salad

Ingredients:

6 to 7 cups endive, 3 bundles, trimmed

1/4 cucumber, halved lengthwise, then thinly
sliced3 tablespoons chopped or snipped chives

16 cherry tomatoes

1/2 cup sliced

almonds1/4 white

onion, sliced

Salt and pepper, to

taste5 ounces ricotta

cheese

3 ounces cheddar cheese , shredded

Dressing

1 sprig cilantro, minced

1 tablespoon distilled white

vinegar 1/4 lemon, juiced, about 2
teaspoons 1/4 cup extra-virgin
olive oil

1 tsp. egg free mayonnaise

Prep

Combine all of the dressing ingredients in a food
processor. Toss with the rest of the ingredients and
combine well.

Mesclun and Romano Cheese Salad

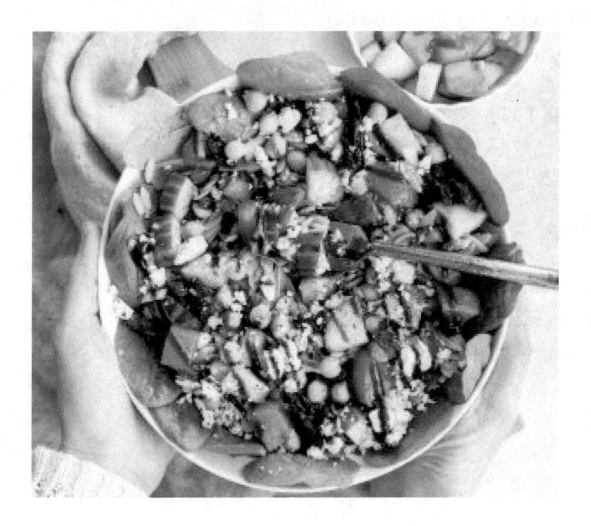

Ingredients:

6 to 7 cups mesclun, 3 bundles, trimmed

¼ zucchini, halved lengthwise, then thinly sliced3 tablespoons chopped or snipped chives

16 cherry tomatoes
1/2 cup sliced

almonds 1/4 white
onion, sliced

Salt and pepper, to taste

3 ounces pecorino romano cheese,
shredded 3 ounces cream cheese,
crumbled

Dressing

1 tablespoon distilled white
vinegar 1/4 lemon, juiced, about 2
teaspoons 1/4 cup extra-virgin
olive oil

1 tsp. pesto sauce

Prep

Combine all of the dressing ingredients in a food
processor. Toss with the rest of the ingredients and
combine well.

Kale Cucumber Tomatillo and Camambert Salad

Ingredients:

6 to 7 cups kale, 3 bundles, trimmed

1/4 cucumber, halved lengthwise, then thinly
sliced 3 tablespoons chopped or snipped chives

16 green tomatillos, sliced in
half 1/2 cup sliced almonds

1/4 white onion, sliced
Salt and pepper, to
taste

3 ounces cream cheese, crumbled

3 ounces camembert cheese, crumbled

Dressing

1 sprig cilantro, minced

1 tablespoon distilled white
vinegar 1/4 lemon, juiced, about 2

teaspoons1/4 cup extra-virgin
olive oil

1 tsp. English mustard

Prep

Combine all of the dressing ingredients in a food processor. Toss with the rest of the ingredients and combine well.

Spinach and Camambert Salad

Ingredients:

6 to 7 cups spinach, 3 bundles, trimmed

1/4 cucumber, halved lengthwise, then thinly
sliced3 tablespoons chopped or snipped chives

16 tomatillos, sliced in
half1/2 cup sliced
almonds 1/4 white
onion, sliced Salt and
pepper, to taste

3 ounces camembert cheese,
crumbled3 ounces mozarella cheese,
shredded

Dressing

1 sprig cilantro, minced

1 tablespoon distilled white
vinegar 1/4 lemon, juiced, about 2

teaspoons 1/4 cup extra-virgin
olive oil

1 tsp. egg free mayonnaise

Prep

Combine all of the dressing ingredients in a food
processor. Toss with the rest of the ingredients and
combine well.

Kale Tomato and Pepperjack Cheese Salad

Ingredients:

6 to 7 cups kale, 3 bundles, trimmed

1/4 cucumber, halved lengthwise, then thinly
sliced 3 tablespoons chopped or snipped chives

16 cherry tomatoes

1/2 cup sliced

almonds 1/4 white

onion, sliced

Salt and pepper, to taste

3 ounces pepperjack cheese, shredded

3 ounces pecorino romano cheese, shredded

Dressing

1 sprig cilantro, minced

1 tablespoon distilled white
vinegar 1/4 lemon, juiced, about 2

teaspoons 1/4 cup extra-virgin olive oil

1 tsp. English mustard

Prep

Combine all of the dressing ingredients in a food processor. Toss with the rest of the ingredients and combine well.

Spinach Tomato and Parmesan Cheese Salad

Ingredients:

6 to 7 cups spinach, 3 bundles, trimmed

1/4 cucumber, halved lengthwise, then thinly
sliced 3 tablespoons chopped or snipped chives

16 cherry tomatoes
1/2 cup sliced
almonds 1/4 white
onion, sliced

Salt and pepper, to taste

3 ounces mozarella cheese,
shredded 6 ounces parmesan
cheese, shredded

Dressing

1 sprig cilantro, minced

1 tablespoon distilled white

vinegar 1/4 lemon, juiced, about 2
teaspoons 1/4 cup extra-virgin
olive oil

1 tsp. English mustard

Prep

Combine all of the dressing ingredients in a food
processor. Toss with the rest of the ingredients and
combine well.

Napa Cabbage Tomatillo and Tofu Ricotta Cheese Salad

Ingredients:

6 to 7 cups napa cabbage, 3 bundles, trimmed

1/4 cucumber, halved lengthwise, then thinly sliced3 tablespoons chopped or snipped chives

16 green tomatillos, sliced in half1/2 cup sliced almonds

1/4 white onion, sliced
Salt and pepper, to
taste

1 ounce blue cheese, crumbled

6 ounces gouda cheese, shredded

Dressing

1 sprig cilantro, minced

1 tablespoon distilled white
vinegar 1/4 lemon, juiced, about 2

teaspoons 1/4 cup extra-virgin
olive oil

1 tsp. egg free mayonnaise

Prep

Combine all of the dressing ingredients in a food
processor. Toss with the rest of the ingredients and
combine well.

Chervil Tomatoes & Almond Salad

Ingredients:

6 to 7 cups chervil, 3 bundles, trimmed

1/4 cucumber, halved lengthwise, then thinly
sliced3 tablespoons chopped or snipped chives

16 cherry tomatoes

1/2 cup sliced

almonds1/4 white

onion, sliced

Salt and pepper, to taste

6 ounces gouda cheese,

shredded3 ounces brie cheese,

crumbled

Dressing

1 sprig cilantro, minced

1 tablespoon distilled white

vinegar 1/4 lemon, juiced, about 2
teaspoons1/4 cup extra-virgin
olive oil

1 tsp. English mustard

Prep

Combine all of the dressing ingredients in a food
processor. Toss with the rest of the ingredients and
combine well.

Bib Lettuce Tomatillo and Vegan Parmesan Cheese Salad

Ingredients:

6 to 7 cups bib lettuce, 3 bundles, trimmed

1/4 cucumber, halved lengthwise, then thinly
sliced 3 tablespoons chopped or snipped chives

16 tomatillos, sliced in
half 1/2 cup sliced
almonds 1/4 white
onion, sliced Salt and
pepper, to taste

7 ounces parmesan cheese,
shredded 1 ounce blue cheese,
crumbled

Dressing

1 sprig cilantro, minced

1 tablespoon distilled white
vinegar 1/4 lemon, juiced, about 2

teaspoons 1/4 cup extra-virgin
olive oil

Prep

Combine all of the dressing ingredients in a food
processor. Toss with the rest of the ingredients and
combine well.

Chicory Tomatillo and Almond Salad

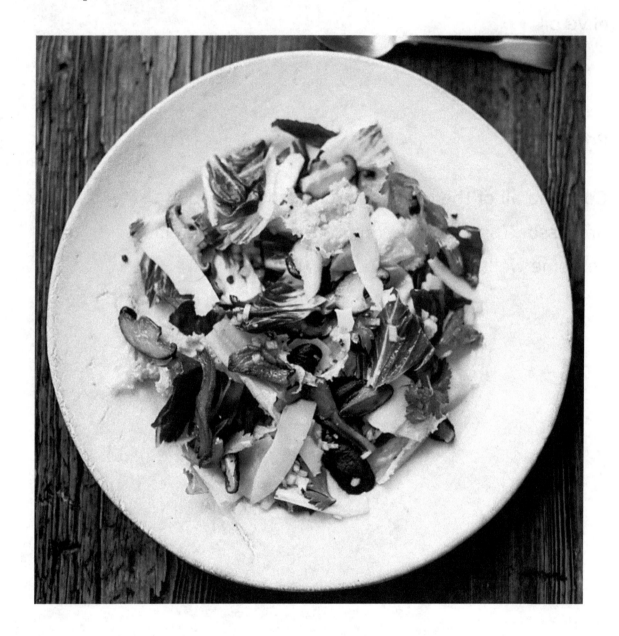

Ingredients:

6 to 7 cups chicory, 3 bundles, trimmed

1/4 cucumber, halved lengthwise, then thinly
sliced 3 tablespoons chopped or snipped chives

16 green tomatillos, sliced in
half1/2 cup sliced almonds

1/4 white onion, sliced
Salt and pepper, to
taste

5 ounces feta cheese, crumbled

3 ounces monterey jack cheese, shredded

Dressing

1 sprig cilantro, minced

1 tablespoon distilled white
vinegar 1/4 lemon, juiced, about 2
teaspoons1/4 cup extra-virgin
olive oil

1 tsp. English mustard

Prep

Combine all of the dressing ingredients in a food

processor. Toss with the rest of the ingredients and combine well.

Baby Beet Greens Tomatoes and Tofu Ricotta Cheese Salad

Ingredients:

6 to 7 cups baby beet greens, 3 bundles,
trimmed 1/4 cucumber, halved lengthwise,
then thinly sliced3 tablespoons chopped or
snipped chives

16 cherry tomatoes
1/2 cup sliced
almonds1/4 white
onion, sliced

Salt and pepper, to taste

3 ounces cheddar cheese ,
shredded5 ounces cottage cheese,
crumbled

Dressing

1 sprig cilantro, minced

1 tablespoon distilled white
vinegar 1/4 lemon, juiced, about 2
teaspoons1/4 cup extra-virgin
olive oil

1 tsp. egg free mayonnaise

Prep

Combine all of the dressing ingredients in a food
processor.Toss with the rest of the ingredients and
combine well.

Napa Cabbage Tomatoes and Cottage Cheese Salad

Ingredients:

6 to 7 cups Napa cabbage, 3 bundles, trimmed

1/4 cucumber, halved lengthwise, then thinly
sliced3 tablespoons chopped or snipped chives

16 cherry tomatoes

1/2 cup sliced

almonds1/4 white

onion, sliced

Salt and pepper, to taste

3 ounces cottage cheese, crumbled

5 ounces pecorino romano cheese, shredded

Dressing

1 sprig cilantro, minced

1 tablespoon distilled white
vinegar 1/4 lemon, juiced, about 2

teaspoons 1/4 cup extra-virgin
olive oil

Prep

Combine all of the dressing ingredients in a food
processor. Toss with the rest of the ingredients and
combine well.

Kale and Cheddar Cheese Salad

Ingredients:

6 to 7 cups kale, 3 bundles, trimmed

1/4 cucumber, halved lengthwise, then thinly
sliced 3 tablespoons chopped or snipped chives

16 tomatillos, sliced in
half 1/2 cup sliced
almonds 1/4 white
onion, sliced Salt and
pepper, to taste

5 ounces monterey jack cheese,
shredded 3 ounces cheddar cheese ,
shredded

Dressing

1 sprig cilantro, minced

1 tablespoon distilled white
vinegar 1/4 lemon, juiced, about 2

teaspoons 1/4 cup extra-virgin
olive oil

1 tsp. English mustard

Prep

Combine all of the dressing ingredients in a food
processor. Toss with the rest of the ingredients and
combine well.

Super Simple Bib Lettuce Salad

Ingredients:

1 head bib lettuce, rinsed, patted and shredded

Dressing

1/2 cup white wine vinegar

1 tablespoon extra virgin olive oilFreshly ground black pepper

3 ounces pecorino romano cheese, shreddedSea salt

Prep

Combine all of the dressing ingredients in a food processor.Toss with the rest of the ingredients and combine well.

Easy Romaine Lettuce Salad

Ingredients:

1 head romaine lettuce, rinsed, patted and shredded

Dressing

2 tbsp. white wine vinegar

4 tablespoons macadamia oil Freshly ground black pepper 3/4 cup finely ground peanutsSea salt

Prep

Combine all of the dressing ingredients in a food processor. Toss with the rest of the ingredients and combine well.

Bib Boston Salad

Ingredients:

1 head bib lettuce, rinsed, patted and shredded

Dressing

2 tbsp. apple cider
vinegar4 tablespoons
olive oil

Freshly ground black pepper

3 ounces gouda cheese,
shreddedSea salt

Prep

Combine all of the dressing ingredients in a food processor.Toss with the rest of the ingredients and combine well.

Conclusion

Unfortunately this wonderful vegetarian cookbook ends here, but don't worry, many more will be coming soon, more and more interesting, stay updated!

If your passion for cooking is strong then I am sure you will have found our curious and exquisite recipes.

at this point, before saying goodbye, we would like to give you an advice, that is, always try to combine a healthy lifestyle with a balanced diet made up of our delicious recipes: this is the best combination. the time has come to say goodbye with a big hug, see you soon with many news.

CPSIA information can be obtained
at www.ICGtesting.com
Printed in the USA
BVHW061226130421
604816BV00004B/901